GW00383419

This portfolio is a tool to help you record your evidence of practice and CPD However the NMC insist you use only their forms for reflective accounts, reflective discussion and the confirmation form. However I have included similar forms in this portfolio for planning and teaching purposes. Please use the NMC website to download the valid forms before submitting your revalidation.

My Revalidation Portfolio© 2016LucyAdams

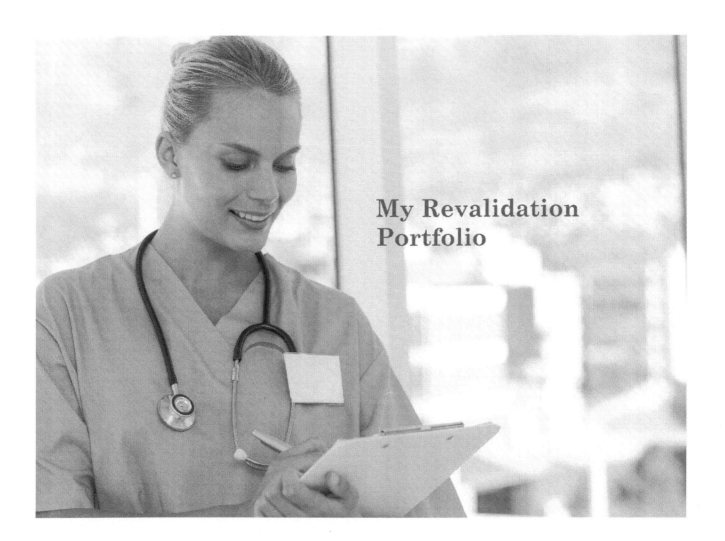

My Revalidation Portfolio

Name...

Telephone Number...

Contents

Evidence of 450 Practice Hours

Date or dates of Practice	Number of Hours worked	Name and address of the organisation	Scope of Practice E.g. Direct patient care	Work Setting E.g. Hospital ward	Brief description of the work you did	Your Registration E.g. Nurse

Evidence of 450 Practice Hours

Date or dates of Practice	Number of Hours worked	Name and address of the organisation	Scope of Practice E.g. Direct patient care	Work Setting E.g. Hospital ward	Brief description of the work you did	Your Registration E.g. Nurse

Evidence of 450 Practice Hours

Date or dates of Practice	Number of Hours worked	Name and address of the organisation	Scope of Practice E.g. Direct patient care	Work Setting E.g. Hospital ward	Brief description of the work you did	Your Registration E.g. Nurse

Evidence of 450 Practice Hours

Date or dates of Practice	Number of Hours worked	Name and address of the organisation	Scope of Practice E.g. Direct patient care	Work Setting E.g. Hospital ward	Brief description of the work you did	Your Registration E.g. Nurse

Evidence of 450 Practice Hours

Date or dates of Practice	Number of Hours worked	Name and address of the organisation	Scope of Practice E.g. Direct patient care	Work Setting E.g. Hospital ward	Brief description of the work you did	Your Registration E.g. Nurse

Evidence of 450 Practice Hours

Date or dates of Practice	Number of Hours worked	Name and address of the organisation	Scope of Practice E.g. Direct patient care	Work Setting E.g. Hospital ward	Brief description of the work you did	Your Registration E.g. Nurse

Evidence of 450 Practice Hours

Date or dates of Practice	Number of Hours worked	Name and address of the organisation	Scope of Practice E.g. Direct patient care	Work Setting E.g. Hospital ward	Brief description of the work you did	Your Registration E.g. Nurse

Evidence of 450 Practice Hours

Date or dates of Practice	Number of Hours worked	Name and address of the organisation	Scope of Practice E.g. Direct patient care	Work Setting E.g. Hospital ward	Brief description of the work you did	Your Registration E.g. Nurse

Evidence of 450 Practice Hours

Date or dates of Practice	Number of Hours worked	Name and address of the organisation	Scope of Practice E.g. Direct patient care	Work Setting E.g. Hospital ward	Brief description of the work you did	Your Registration E.g. Nurse

Evidence of 450 Practice Hours

Date or dates of Practice	Number of Hours worked	Name and address of the organisation	Scope of Practice E.g. Direct patient care	Work Setting E.g. Hospital ward	Brief description of the work you did	Your Registration E.g. Nurse

Evidence of 450 Practice Hours

Date or dates of Practice	Number of Hours worked	Name and address of the organisation	Scope of Practice E.g. Direct patient care	Work Setting E.g. Hospital ward	Brief description of the work you did	Your Registration E.g. Nurse

Evidence of 450 Practice Hours

Date or dates of Practice	Number of Hours worked	Name and address of the organisation	Scope of Practice E.g. Direct patient care	Work Setting E.g. Hospital ward	Brief description of the work you did	Your Registration E.g. Nurse

Evidence of 450 Practice Hours

Date or dates of Practice	Number of Hours worked	Name and address of the organisation	Scope of Practice E.g. Direct patient care	Work Setting E.g. Hospital ward	Brief description of the work you did	Your Registration E.g. Nurse

Evidence of 450 Practice Hours

Date or dates of Practice	Number of Hours worked	Name and address of the organisation	Scope of Practice E.g. Direct patient care	Work Setting E.g. Hospital ward	Brief description of the work you did	Your Registration E.g. Nurse

Evidence of 450 Practice Hours

Date or dates of Practice	Number of Hours worked	Name and address of the organisation	Scope of Practice E.g. Direct patient care	Work Setting E.g. Hospital ward	Brief description of the work you did	Your Registration E.g. Nurse

Evidence of 450 Practice Hours

Date or dates of Practice	Number of Hours worked	Name and address of the organisation	Scope of Practice E.g. Direct patient care	Work Setting E.g. Hospital ward	Brief description of the work you did	Your Registration E.g. Nurse

Evidence of 450 Practice Hours

Date or dates of Practice	Number of Hours worked	Name and address of the organisation	Scope of Practice E.g. Direct patient care	Work Setting E.g. Hospital ward	Brief description of the work you did	Your Registration E.g. Nurse

Evidence of 450 Practice Hours

Date or dates of Practice	Number of Hours worked	Name and address of the organisation	Scope of Practice E.g. Direct patient care	Work Setting E.g. Hospital ward	Brief description of the work you did	Your Registration E.g. Nurse

Evidence of 450 Practice Hours

Date or dates of Practice	Number of Hours worked	Name and address of the organisation	Scope of Practice E.g. Direct patient care	Work Setting E.g. Hospital ward	Brief description of the work you did	Your Registration E.g. Nurse

Evidence of 450 Practice Hours

Date or dates of Practice	Number of Hours worked	Name and address of the organisation	Scope of Practice E.g. Direct patient care	Work Setting E.g. Hospital ward	Brief description of the work you did	Your Registration E.g. Nurse

Evidence of 450 Practice Hours

Date or dates of Practice	Number of Hours worked	Name and address of the organisation	Scope of Practice E.g. Direct patient care	Work Setting E.g. Hospital ward	Brief description of the work you did	Your Registration E.g. Nurse

Evidence of 450 Practice Hours

Date or dates of Practice	Number of Hours worked	Name and address of the organisation	Scope of Practice E.g. Direct patient care	Work Setting E.g. Hospital ward	Brief description of the work you did	Your Registration E.g. Nurse

Evidence of 450 Practice Hours

Date or dates of Practice	Number of Hours worked	Name and address of the organisation	Scope of Practice E.g. Direct patient care	Work Setting E.g. Hospital ward	Brief description of the work you did	Your Registration E.g. Nurse

Evidence of 450 Practice Hours

Date or dates of Practice	Number of Hours worked	Name and address of the organisation	Scope of Practice E.g. Direct patient care	Work Setting E.g. Hospital ward	Brief description of the work you did	Your Registration E.g. Nurse

Evidence of 450 Practice Hours

Date or dates of Practice	Number of Hours worked	Name and address of the organisation	Scope of Practice E.g. Direct patient care	Work Setting E.g. Hospital ward	Brief description of the work you did	Your Registration E.g. Nurse

Evidence of 450 Practice Hours

Date or dates of Practice	Number of Hours worked	Name and address of the organisation	Scope of Practice E.g. Direct patient care	Work Setting E.g. Hospital ward	Brief description of the work you did	Your Registration E.g. Nurse

Evidence of 450 Practice Hours

Date or dates of Practice	Number of Hours worked	Name and address of the organisation	Scope of Practice E.g. Direct patient care	Work Setting E.g. Hospital ward	Brief description of the work you did	Your Registration E.g. Nurse

Evidence of 450 Practice Hours

Date or dates of Practice	Number of Hours worked	Name and address of the organisation	Scope of Practice E.g. Direct patient care	Work Setting E.g. Hospital ward	Brief description of the work you did	Your Registration E.g. Nurse

Evidence of 450 Practice Hours

Date or dates of Practice	Number of Hours worked	Name and address of the organisation	Scope of Practice E.g. Direct patient care	Work Setting E.g. Hospital ward	Brief description of the work you did	Your Registration E.g. Nurse

Evidence of 450 Practice Hours

Date or dates of Practice	Number of Hours worked	Name and address of the organisation	Scope of Practice E.g. Direct patient care	Work Setting E.g. Hospital ward	Brief description of the work you did	Your Registration E.g. Nurse

Continuing Professional Development Log

Evidence of 35 hours study including 20 hours participatory learning

Date	Method	Topic	Link to Code	Individual Hours	Participatory Hours

Continuing Professional Development Log
Evidence of 35 hours study including 20 hours participatory learning

Date	Method	Topic	Link to Code	Individual Hours	Participatory Hours

Continuing Professional Development Log

Evidence of 35 hours study including 20 hours participatory learning

Date	Method	Topic	Link to Code	Individual Hours	Participatory Hours

Continuing Professional Development Log

Evidence of 35 hours study including 20 hours participatory learning

Date	Method	Topic	Link to Code	Individual Hours	Participatory Hours

Continuing Professional Development Log

Evidence of 35 hours study including 20 hours participatory learning

Date	Method	Topic	Link to Code	Individual Hours	Participatory Hours

Continuing Professional Development Log

Evidence of 35 hours study including 20 hours participatory learning

Date	Method	Topic	Link to Code	Individual Hours	Participatory Hours

Reflective Accounts

Please note these forms are for planning purposes only. Before submitting to NMC please download their forms from their website.

Type of Reflective account	
What did you learn from the CPD activity and/or feedback and/or event or experience in your practice?	
How did you change or improve your practice as a result?	
Relevance to the code	

Reflective Accounts

Please note these forms are for planning purposes only. Before submitting to NMC please download their forms from their website.

Type of Reflective account	
What did you learn from the CPD activity and/or feedback and/or event or experience in your practice?	
How did you change or improve your practice as a result?	
Relevance to the code	

Reflective Accounts

Please note these forms are for planning purposes only. Before submitting to NMC please download their forms from their website.

Type of Reflective account	
What did you learn from the CPD activity and/or feedback and/or event or experience in your practice?	
How did you change or improve your practice as a result?	
Relevance to the code	

Reflective Accounts

Please note these forms are for planning purposes only. Before submitting to NMC please download their forms from their website.

Type of Reflective account	
What did you learn from the CPD activity and/or feedback and/or event or experience in your practice?	
How did you change or improve your practice as a result?	
Relevance to the code	

Reflective Accounts

Please note these forms are for planning purposes only. Before submitting to NMC please download their forms from their website.

Type of Reflective account	
What did you learn from the CPD activity and/or feedback and/or event or experience in your practice?	
How did you change or improve your practice as a result?	
Relevance to the code	

Reflective Accounts

Please note these forms are for planning purposes only. Before submitting to NMC please download their forms from their website.

Type of Reflective account	
What did you learn from the CPD activity and/or feedback and/or event or experience in your practice?	
How did you change or improve your practice as a result?	
Relevance to the code	

Reflective Accounts

Please note these forms are for planning purposes only. Before submitting to NMC please download their forms from their website.

Type of Reflective account	
What did you learn from the CPD activity and/or feedback and/or event or experience in your practice?	
How did you change or improve your practice as a result?	
Relevance to the code	

Reflective Accounts

Please note these forms are for planning purposes only. Before submitting to NMC please download their forms from their website.

Type of Reflective account	
What did you learn from the CPD activity and/or feedback and/or event or experience in your practice?	
How did you change or improve your practice as a result?	
Relevance to the code	

Reflective Accounts

Please note these forms are for planning purposes only. Before submitting to NMC please download their forms from their website.

Type of Reflective account	
What did you learn from the CPD activity and/or feedback and/or event or experience in your practice?	
How did you change or improve your practice as a result?	
Relevance to the code	

Reflective Accounts

Please note these forms are for planning purposes only. Before submitting to NMC please download their forms from their website.

Type of Reflective account	
What did you learn from the CPD activity and/or feedback and/or event or experience in your practice?	
How did you change or improve your practice as a result?	
Relevance to the code	

Relective Discussion Form

Please note these forms are for planning purposes only. Before submitting to NMC please download their forms from their website.

Your Name;	
Your NMC Pin;	
Name of Nurse or Midwife involved in discussion;	
Their NMC Pin	
Their Email Address;	
Their work Address including Postcode;	
Their Contact Telephone Number	
Date of Discussion;	
Summary of discussion;	
I have discussed five written reflective accounts with the named nurse or midwife as part of a reflective discussion. I agree to be contacted by the NMC to provide further information if necessary for verification purposes.	Signature; Date;

Relective Discussion Form

Please note these forms are for planning purposes only. Before submitting to NMC please download their forms from their website.

Your Name;	
Your NMC Pin;	
Name of Nurse or Midwife involved in discussion;	
Their NMC Pin	
Their Email Address;	
Their work Address including Postcode;	
Their Contact Telephone Number	
Date of Discussion;	
Summary of discussion;	
I have discussed five written reflective accounts with the named nurse or midwife as part of a reflective discussion. I agree to be contacted by the NMC to provide further information if necessary for verification purposes.	Signature; Date;

Relective Discussion Form

Please note these forms are for planning purposes only. Before submitting to NMC please download their forms from their website.

Your Name;	
Your NMC Pin;	
Name of Nurse or Midwife involved in discussion;	
Their NMC Pin	
Their Email Address;	
Their work Address including Postcode;	
Their Contact Telephone Number	
Date of Discussion;	
Summary of discussion;	

I have discussed five written reflective accounts with the named nurse or midwife as part of a reflective discussion. I agree to be contacted by the NMC to provide further information if necessary for verification purposes.	Signature; Date;

Relective Discussion Form

Please note these forms are for planning purposes only. Before submitting to NMC please download their forms from their website.

Your Name;	
Your NMC Pin;	
Name of Nurse or Midwife involved in discussion;	
Their NMC Pin	
Their Email Address;	
Their work Address including Postcode;	
Their Contact Telephone Number	
Date of Discussion;	
Summary of discussion;	
I have discussed five written reflective accounts with the named nurse or midwife as part of a reflective discussion. I agree to be contacted by the NMC to provide further information if necessary for verification purposes.	Signature; Date;

Confirmation Form

Please note this form can be used for planning purposes. Before submitting to NMC please download their confirmation form.

To be completed by the nurse or midwife:

Name:	
NMC Pin:	
Date of last renewal of registration or joined the register:	

I have received confirmation from (select applicable):

☐	A line manager who is also an NMC-registered nurse or midwife
☐	Another NMC registered nurse or midwife
☐	A regulated healthcare professional
☐	An overseas regulated healthcare professional
☐	Other professionals in accordance with the NMC online confirmation tool

To be completed by the confirmer:

Name:	
Job title:	
Email address:	
Work address including postcode:	
Contact number:	
Date of confirmation discussion:	

If you are an NMC-registered nurse or midwife please provide:

NMC Pin:

If you are a regulated healthcare professional please provide:

Profession:
Registration number for regulatory body:

If you are an overseas regulated healthcare professional please provide:

Country:	
Profession:	
Registration number for regulatory body:	

If you are another professional please provide:

Profession:	
Registration number for regulatory body (if relevant):	

Confirmation checklist of revalidation requirements

Practice hours

☐ You have seen written evidence that satisfies you that the nurse or midwife has practised the minimum number of hours required for their registration.

Continuing professional development

☐ You have seen written evidence that satisfies you that the nurse or midwife has undertaken 35 hours of CPD relevant to their practice as a nurse or midwife

☐ You have seen evidence that at least 20 of the 35 hours include participatory learning relevant to their practice as a nurse or midwife.

☐ You have seen accurate records of the CPD undertaken.

Practice-related feedback

☐ You are satisfied that the nurse or midwife has obtained five pieces of practice-related feedback.

Written reflective accounts

☐ You have seen five written reflective accounts on the nurse or midwife's CPD and/or practice-related feedback and/or an event or experience in their practice and how this relates to the Code, recorded on the NMC form.

Reflective discussion

☐ You have seen a completed and signed form showing that the nurse or midwife has discussed their reflective accounts with another NMC-registered nurse or midwife (or you are an NMC-registered nurse or midwife who has discussed these with the nurse or midwife yourself).

I confirm that I have read 'Information for confirmers', and that the above named NMC-registered nurse or midwife has demonstrated to me that they have complied with all of the NMC revalidation requirements listed above over the three years since their registration was last renewed or they joined the register as set out in 'Information for confirmers'.

I agree to be contacted by the NMC to provide further information if necessary for verification purposes. I am aware that if I do not respond to a request for verification information I may put the nurse or midwife's revalidation application at risk.

Signature:

Date:

Confirmation Form

Please note this form can be used for planning purposes. Before submitting to NMC please download their confirmation form.

To be completed by the nurse or midwife:

Name:	
NMC Pin:	
Date of last renewal of registration or joined the register:	

I have received confirmation from (select applicable):

☐	A line manager who is also an NMC-registered nurse or midwife
☐	Another NMC registered nurse or midwife
☐	A regulated healthcare professional
☐	An overseas regulated healthcare professional
☐	Other professionals in accordance with the NMC online confirmation tool

To be completed by the confirmer:

Name:	
Job title:	
Email address:	
Work address including postcode:	
Contact number:	
Date of confirmation discussion:	

If you are an NMC-registered nurse or midwife please provide:

NMC Pin:

If you are a regulated healthcare professional please provide:

Profession:
Registration number for regulatory body:

If you are an overseas regulated healthcare professional please provide:

Country:
Profession:
Registration number for regulatory body:

If you are another professional please provide:

Profession:
Registration number for regulatory body (if relevant):

Confirmation checklist of revalidation requirements

Practice hours

☐ You have seen written evidence that satisfies you that the nurse or midwife has practised the minimum number of hours required for their registration.

Continuing professional development

☐ You have seen written evidence that satisfies you that the nurse or midwife has undertaken 35 hours of CPD relevant to their practice as a nurse or midwife

☐ You have seen evidence that at least 20 of the 35 hours include participatory learning relevant to their practice as a nurse or midwife.

☐ You have seen accurate records of the CPD undertaken.

Practice-related feedback

☐ You are satisfied that the nurse or midwife has obtained five pieces of practice-related feedback.

Written reflective accounts

☐ You have seen five written reflective accounts on the nurse or midwife's CPD and/or practice-related feedback and/or an event or experience in their practice and how this relates to the Code, recorded on the NMC form.

Reflective discussion

☐ You have seen a completed and signed form showing that the nurse or midwife has discussed their reflective accounts with another NMC-registered nurse or midwife (or you are an NMC-registered nurse or midwife who has discussed these with the nurse or midwife yourself).

I confirm that I have read 'Information for confirmers', and that the above named NMC-registered nurse or midwife has demonstrated to me that they have complied with all of the NMC revalidation requirements listed above over the three years since their registration was last renewed or they joined the register as set out in 'Information for confirmers'.

I agree to be contacted by the NMC to provide further information if necessary for verification purposes. I am aware that if I do not respond to a request for verification information I may put the nurse or midwife's revalidation application at risk.

Signature:

Date:

Notes

Notes

Notes

Notes

Notes

Notes

Notes

Notes

Notes

Notes

Notes

Notes

Notes

Notes

Notes

Printed in Great Britain
by Amazon